Clara Brown

The Inside Truth

About Nursing Homes

outskirts
press

The Inside Truth About Nursing Homes
All Rights Reserved.
Copyright © 2019 Clara Brown
v1.0

The opinions expressed in this manuscript are solely the opinions of the author and do not represent the opinions or thoughts of the publisher. The author has represented and warranted full ownership and/or legal right to publish all the materials in this book.

This book may not be reproduced, transmitted, or stored in whole or in part by any means, including graphic, electronic, or mechanical without the express written consent of the publisher except in the case of brief quotations embodied in critical articles and reviews.

Outskirts Press, Inc.
http://www.outskirtspress.com

ISBN: 978-1-9772-0981-8

Cover Photo © 2019 www.gettyimages.com. All rights reserved - used with permission.

Outskirts Press and the "OP" logo are trademarks belonging to Outskirts Press, Inc.

PRINTED IN THE UNITED STATES OF AMERICA

THIS BOOK WAS WRITTEN BY MARY F, BRAKE AND CLARA L. BROWN

IN 1978. THIS BOOK WAS WRITTEN TO LET PEOPLE KNOW THE TRUTH ABOUT NURSING HOMES. THIS BOOK IS DEDICATED TO MY MOTHER MARY F. BRAKE WHO HAS GONE TO BE WITH OUR LORD.

          MARY F. BRAKE
            AND
         CLARA L. ALLENBROWN

Table of Contents

Chapter 1 1

Chapter 2 9

Chapter 3 18

Chapter 4 29

Chapter 5 39

Chapter 1
The Inside Truth About Nursing Homes

My daughter and i have spent many years working in nursing homes.

We have seen a lot of terrible thing that goes on in nursing homes.

These old people that are put in these homes and are forgotten about. these old people are at the mercy of the owners and the nursing staff.

My daughter and I decided to write this book. We are going to tell the whole truth about what really goes on in these places.

These stories are all true. Not even one is a lie. People can just read these stories, then they might think twice before putting their parents, grandparents, or aunts and uncles in these places.

When my daughter and I wrote this book, they didn't have men nurses, but now they do and that makes it even more worse for the old people. You won't believe what you are about to read.

Mom and I wrote this book back in the 70's. The first page was lost so I had to rewrite the first page. Mom is gone now but I know one thing. She never had to go to a nursing home.

I will be finishing this book for mom. I know that is what she would have wanted me to do. The stories are all true.

When applying for state license the wiring had to be inspected.

Fine! But now how often after that is the wiring inspected? Then comes the heating and plumbing. How closely after the first inspection are these inspected and how often? If these were inspected very closely at least once a year maybe there wouldn't be so many fires and so many old people's lives lost. Faulty wiring, faulty furnaces and flues can easily cause tragedy to a nursing homes.

After reading in the papers about two nursing homes in a period of one year in the state of Ohio where several old people were burned to death I think it is time to start thinking. I feel the states should be more critical and severe in their inspections and more often.

When the building is old and an application is made for a license the first thing the state inspection should do is closely inspect the wiring and the heating. If the furnace is old even though it works it should be replaced with a new one. This seems cruel and cynical but many old peoples lives are in the owners hands then let them invest the money to have the home in first class conditions.

One thing that I fully believe should not be allowed is repair work becoming a patch up job, or using second hand material and also letting just anyone do the work. There are a lot of people who knows how to install or repair a furnace or set in a receptiable but because of the responsibility all this should be done by a reliable licensed repairman. I am sure most of you who may read this will agree with me. If anyone of you dear readers where to place one of your loved ones in a nursing home, wouldn't you feel more at ease to know that the furnace was in A-1 condition and the wiring was in excellent condition? Well this has a lot to do with a lot of fires today.

Now let's talk about the help. This too is a very important factor. The state law is only a licensed practical nurse or a registered nurse be allowed to give the old people medicine.

But this law is not enforced in most of the nursing homes. I have never worked in a nursing home in all my years that this rule was carried out to the tee. Also a lock is to be on medicine cabinets and it is to be locked at all times. This too is not carried out. Unless the one that give out the medicine is licensed it is the same as the heating and wiring.

As we go on in this writing I will point out to you the examples of the damage that can be done by just anyone giving out medicine to old people . If an aid wants to learn medicine and wants to become a licensed practical nurse, let her get her training in a hospital. Not in a nursing home. In most any hospital there is a nurses training course where can work while you are in training.

The help in the nursing home is very unreliable. It seems the operators hire young girls that work for only two things, quitting time and payday. They do not care about the old people. The young girls do not have the patience with the old people.

If an old person is very senile and does a lot of roaming around the girl grows impatient. She becomes irritable with the old person and sometimes become very mean to them. This may not be so in some young aides.

But dear readers it is so in most cases.

She will jerk the old person around and the first thing that comes to her mind is restrainers. She'll tie the poor old person to the bed and give her a sleeping pill or a shot.

This i say is the owners fault. In the first place the owner should be sure the young lady they hired was kind , patient, and understanding. But the owner doesn't have the welfare of their old people at heart. If they did they would be more careful who they hired.

Let's go back to the aides giving out the medicine. Here is a true example of what really goes on in nursing homes.

Mrs. Smith, Mrs. Woods and Mrs. Roberts all share the same room. A young aide whom we shall call Polly working on the second shift. She is alone. It is time for the bedtime medicine, and Polly wants to get the medicine given so she can make some phone calls. Even though the medicine was put in the little cups on a card on a tray. Polly has other things on her mind. She gives Mrs. Woods the pill that should be given to Mrs. Roberts. Mrs. Woods becomes ill because of this mistake. Polly has given out the medicine and is on the phone. Mrs. Woods calls and calls but Polly doesn't hear her because she is busy talking on the phone. By the time the third shift girl comes in at 11:00 P.M. , Mrs.

Woods is in need of a doctor. No one knows what happened. The third shift girl calls the owner and they send Mrs. Woods to the hospital where it is found the wrong medicine was given.

My Dear readers I know this is true because i have seen it happen many times. Maybe Mrs. Woods doesn't die but through negligence on the owner of the nursing home an old person has became very ill.

In the first place dear readers, there should be a licensed Practical nurse and an aide on the second and third shifts. There are usually three besides the owner on the first shift. Where there are fifteen or more patients in a nursing home that is licensed there should always be an L.P.N. (Licensed Practical Nurse) on duty with the aide on the last two shifts. But many nursing homes have only one nurse and that is just an aide. This law should be enforced before licenses are issued.

The people who own and operate a nursing home are really the blame for all the things that goes on unseen in the nursing homes of today. Why?

Well let's talk about it. Let's talk about the wages and conditions under which the girls work. The wages are very low. If any aide gets $1.65 an hour in the state of Ohio and most states in the midwest they are getting top wages. This is very unfair because this kind of work is hard work. The nurses have to do dishes, mop floors, give baths, shave men, do the laundry, including the ironing. They have all the heavy lifting to do and most help does the cooking. The fringe benefits are nothing either. They don't give a vacation with pay. There is no insurance for the help. This too is very unfair.

When a person puts their loved ones in a nursing home the price is high.

Any owner of a licensed nursing home get good money and gets by on the least they can. There should always be a man on duty in case an old person should fall. There should be a woman to do the cleaning and the laundry.

If an owner of a nursing home doesn't clear from fifty to seventy five dollars per month from each old person they want to cut down on the help and make the work load bigger on the help they do keep.

This is true my dear readers. There is very good money in the nursing home business but the way they are operated for the price the old people pay it is really pathetic. The demand for nurses is great and is very good profession but the way nursing homes are operated it is a shame to society.

Now let's talk about the food. It is a shame the way the old people are fed in nursing homes. The old people gets good dinner on Sundays. But the rest of the week the meals are very poor. The reason I speak so plainly dear readers is because I know. After twenty seven years in many different nursing homes I can back up what I have written.

If the state would have investigate more closely and talk to the old people, they would sure have a different opinion on nursing homes.

Whenever the state investigators notify the owner first, If they would just come without notice they would see for themselves what really goes on. They put the best on when they know the inspectors are coming. I have known the inspectors to come and only stay a half hour and of course on the surface everything was fine.

Because a person is put in a nursing home doesn't mean they are too senile to tell what really goes on.

There are a lot of them that would tell many things and speak the truth if they would be spoken too privately but this never happens. But it should. Believe me ! It is no wonder old people have a fear of going to a nursing home.

An old person that is on welfare really get the treatment. Of course there is a T.V. room and a place to sit and read but what about the old people that can't see to read or watch T.V.? Where is the compassion and love for that old person? It doesn't come from the owners and it doesn't come from the help. Oh yes there may be one or two nurses that care but not very many.

I know that there are some old people that are very cruel and very hard to get along with but in my experience with old people I found out that those are the ones that need love more than the others. If a nurse is good to them and they like her they are not very apt to be mean to her.

If the owner of the nursing home would show a little affection toward the old people and they had the feeling that someone cares about them, it gives them a much different outlook on life. This is what old people need is to be wanted, and to know that someone cares. a little bit of kindness on anyone's part to an old person will sure never do any harm.

Stop and think dear readers when have you ever heard any old person say they loved the nursing home they were put in to stay. In most cases after an old person is placed in a nursing home they become most despondent and it is obvious that they feel the bottom had fallen out of their world. What can we do you may say when you read this. Well my dear readers, the one thing and the most important thing that we can do is be very careful where we place them.

If it is impossible to keep our loved ones with us then let us check and recheck the nursing home where we place our loved ones.

There are many private homes that takes old people. Of course some of them are like nursing homes. But as a rule these are some very nice private homes where our loved ones can have love.

When an individual decides they want to own and operate a license nursing home then that is their full time job. They cannot work elsewheres and when they open it up and get old people in all they have to do is to be sure that they are well cared for.

It is their duty to be on twenty four hour call. In a lot of cases a man and his wife run the home.

it is the duty of the operators to check the patients before they leave the home. No one expects them to stay around the clock in the home. But if they would only take the old people's welfare to heart and pay more attention to the old people, nursing homes would be a wonderful thing.

But the way they are operated today it really is heartbreaking.

I will tell you of an incident in a nursing home in Ohio. The lady we shall call her Mrs. Lang, weight 210 pounds. When she was put in the nursing home the owner and operator was a middle aged woman weighing about 185 pounds. Mrs, Lang looked everyday for her son to

The Inside Truth About Nursing Homes

come and see her. He came but not that often. Maybe once a month or maybe every two weeks. At any rate Mrs. Lang would cry because her son didn't come. When the noon meal was served she didn't want to eat. She was despondent and depressed. The owner would slap her and would hold her head back and cram the food into her mouth. It would be the same thing at the evening meal.

I know there was a better way to get that old lady to eat without being so cruel to her. By the end of her first year in the nursing home, she lost weight down to 89 pounds. Would it not have been better dear readers if that owner would of talked nice to that old lady and told her maybe her son was busy working overtime and would come see her as soon as he could. But n she had to be hateful and abusive. No one knows until they work in the nursing home just what really goes on inside of one.

On the rare occasion when the son did come to bring the check, the owner came in all smiles, calling the old lady Honey and patting her hand. This is what really gets to you is this two faced people that operate these nursing homes. The only reason they operate them in the first place dear readers, is that money.

In this same nursing home an old man got out of bed one night and fell and broke his hip. He laid for two days without attention. His daughter came to see him twice a day and when she came she had him taken to the hospital. And it was there she found out he had a broken hip and had it broken for two days.

In another nursing home in Ohio an old man in his late eighties did quite a bit of walking. In mid winter at three A.M. in the morning the old gentleman got out of bed, put on his hat with no coat and walked out of the nursing home. He was found half frozen in just his pajamas around eight A.M.. The police were notified around seven A.M.. There was only one side on and the real question is, "Where was she that she didn't hear the door open and shut?" Another Question was, " Why wasn't all the doors locked?"

In another nursing home in the state of Ohio was a lady around fifty years old. Her mental capacity was very low but she wanted attention. She wanted to be loved and wanted.

Down the hall from her room was another gentleman just a little older. The lady was found in the man's room in the act of love making. Both were in their night clothes. . What Happen to the lady? She was beaten with a spatula, slapped in the face, her T.V. was removed from her room. The man was placed under lock and key for several weeks not being allowed to see anyone.

Now dear readers we all know that these two people needed punishment but not this way. In the first place men and women should not be allowed to be on the same floor, at least so close together. But I feel sure there could of been another way of punishment without brutality. Beating old people is very prominent in nursing homes.

In another nursing home in Ohio, an elderly lady in her early eighties was asked by the owner to leave the nursing home.

The old lady walking with a cane came down the street going to a nursing home about three blocks away. The owner watched and knew where she was going then called the nursing home, gave her a bad reputation and when the old lady finally made it down there the nursing home proprietor told her there was no vacancies.

She started back home, worried and down hearted. A lady sitting on the front porch and saw the old lady come down the street and then saw her come back. She went down to the side walk and talked to the old lady. She was told the nursing home told her to find her a place to go and she would have to do it on her own. The lady asked her about her relatives and she said she had no one.

The lady brought the poor old lady up on the porch. The old lady cried because she didn't know what to do. The lady told her she would take her and she agreed to come. The lady sent a car with a friend to the nursing home, got her belongings and gave her a home.

The owner of the nursing home told the lady " I quote. " You'll be sorry you ever took that old bitty. You won't have her over a month." They told the lady how mean and hateful the old woman was, but you know dear readers the old lady is still living and is still with the lady that took her. This has been seven and one half years ago.

Chapter 2

THIS IS TRUE dear readers because I am the one that took the old lady and I still have her. This occured on June 12, 1964. The old lady was a cook and had owned two large restaurants of her own in Columbus Ohio. I let her go into my kitchen and prepare food. She was very clean. I would tell her she was my right hand. This made her happy and gave her the feeling of being wanted. Today the old lady is almost blind, and has to use a walker. But I would never give her up. If she hears me say I have a headache she will worry over me. She has no one but me dear readers and I have given her happiness and a desire to live. Her mind isn't as good as it was but she can still remember a lot of things. I will really miss her when she is gone. She will be 87 April 23 and I have never forgotten her birthday once since she has been with me. So you see my friends I took an old lady off the street and made her feel wanted and needed. I am happy because i made an old person happy.

Another incident in Ohio nursing home was an old gentleman. For the noon meal the proprietor cooked beef heart and beans. The heart was half cooked and she didn't take the time to cute it for him. He had to be fed and she was cramming it in his mouth very fast. The old man got choked on the half cooked heart and almost choked to death. He had begun to turn blue. She was scared and called for help. They hit the old man in the back and a big piece of the meat flew out onto the floor. He did not want anymore to eat but she made him eat all that was on his plate. She talked very mean to him and told him he could not go out on the porch for a week because he got choked. Tell me my friends was that right? Of course not. Had he had the proper food in the first place, had it been well cooked and had she fed him slowly he would not of chocked. Right?

In another nursing home in Ohio the home was operated by two sisters. One day the furnace went bad and it was very cold. While waiting for the repair man an old lady who walked a lot came to the door of the kitchen and asked why the home was so cold. The owner screamed at her, shoved her back into her room and told her to stay there. When the furnace was repaired the bill was very high. She was angry because of the price she had to pay for the furnace and she cut down on the food for the old people. Those sisters would take turns about going on vacation. They would stay as long as six to eight weeks. They paid very little attention to their old people. The one sister drank quite a lot. But this is another sample of what goes on in nursing homes.

In another nursing home the old people smoked a lot. When they were put to bed some of them would get up in the night and smoked. One night an old man fell asleep and his cigarette dropped from his hand and burned a big hole in the blankets. The owner got so angry she slapped the old man in the face, took his cigarettes away permanently. It was not the old man's life she was interested in but the blankets he ruined. That could of caused a terrible fire and many lives of others.

Where if the owner had been interested in the welfare of her old people she would of taken their cigarettes away at night and gave them back in the morning. She would of had her blankets undamaged and the old people would not of minded to much. So you see dear readers again the owner is at fault.

Another thing that has puzzled me is why things like this never gets into the papers.

All the beatings, starving of these old people, no one seems interested enough to write about it. Even the help won't talk. But I feel it

The Inside Truth About Nursing Homes

is time that someone spoke up. After two big fires and old people getting burned up it is time someone talked. Something has to be done about these nursing homes or God only knows what will happen next.

In each experience I have told you about are true because I was working in them at the time they happened.

I have known my dear readers many old people to cry because they were hungry. Whenever a person can take one half pound of bacon and a dozen of eggs, and feed thirty two people, you know they can not have enough to eat. There have been several nursing homes closed in Ohio because of starving and cruelty to old people.

Here is one experience I'll never be able to forget. It was a lovely nursing home and was operated by a woman. She was so mean to her patients. She beat them, and she came to the point where she wouldn't clean the home up. She wouldn't put out the money for help. One day she just walked away and left twenty eight old people, some invalids alone in the nursing home. They were alone without food for two days until one of them had a visitor and found them in starving condition. Some had wet the bed and wet themselves and some had sat in a chair because they couldn't get up alone. The visitor immediately called the authorities and the old people we placed in another nursing home. I have often wondered how that woman could lie down and sleep. To my knowledge the woman was never found. This has been quite a few years ago. Today there is a nursing home there again but I have never been in it, but knowing the people I feel it's run like many of the others.

Another thing that makes it very hard on many old people is their children. They place the old people in the nursing home and then forget about them. Many children just mail the monthly check and ask about the old people, but never come to see them.

It is a heartbreaking situation to see old person wait and watch and walk and keep asking if their son or daughter had come or called. This is where the old person needs love and understanding most of all.

Most old people have had homes and the children have gotten them after they place the old person in a nursing home. This has caused many old person to go over the deep end. Loneliness for their children. In talking to some other girls that I have worked in nursing homes I was given this information. This comes from checking with other people who have worked in nursing homes for over a period of years and really know the inside of a nursing home.

One girl told me she was working in a nursing home in Ohio and there was an old lady, a very sweet old lady but she loved to sing. She had a tiny doll that she rocked and sang to all day long.

The owner said she (old lady) got on her nerves with the doll and sang to much. She gave her chlorine hydrate and Thorazine and gave her to much. A time the old lady was dead. In the same nursing home later under different management, there was an old man . The old man thought the two old men were intruding and the old man got some server cuts. The owner would not take him to the hospital because she was afraid of the scandal and it would be in the newspapers. The old man was six foot one inch tall. The owner made him sleep in the office on a tiny couch much to short for the old man. He would be so cramped and tired when he got up the next morning he could hardly get around.

He would beg to owner to let him go to his room and sleep in his bed but she said no.

My dear reader you don't know what really go on in the licensed nursing home unless you work in one. Our old people are sadly mistreated and uncared for.

The food is terrible in nursing homes and the old people have to eat it. No wonder so many old people go berserk and are hard to get along with. They are slapped. They are shook. They are tied to chairs and beds. Now would you say this is a good place to put our loved ones? I'm sure you wouldn't.

If the children would be just a little more particular where they placed their loved ones and would listen to the old people when they tell them things that happen maybe these nursing homes could be made more comfortable place for our old people. Also if the state would check just a little close and as I said before talk to some of the old people in private and listen to what they tell them I feel sure this would help a lot. There is a private home in Ohio that has at least four old people or more. She is very hateful with them. The food isn't to bad but the cruelty is terrible.

There is an old woman that wants so bad to get away. But she wont let her out of the yard. She won't allow her to have any company, only her son who is mental. He really isn't capable of making any decisions. He is married and he has a little child. Along with being on the mental side he is very lazy.

He never works and the lady bribes him to say he wants his mother to stay there. She never gets to see anyone but her son. She never gives her old people a cent out of their checks.

It was turned into the Humane Society about her being so cruel to this one old lady.

To my knowledge the man never came to see her. She is the most saddest and unhappy old soul anyone has ever saw. It was also taken up with the welfare department but nothing ever was done about it. The owner tells the old lady if she doesn't say she was happy there, she would be put in a nursing home under restrainers. Now dear readers tell me, is this right? Of course it isn't. If an old person is unhappy where they are and feel they are mistreated the should be allowed to leave. The old lady is just the same as being in prison in solitary confinement.

When the owner gets angry, she has the most vile tongue of any human being. Yet the state lets her have these old people. The Welfare will tell you they want the old people to be happy but when it is reported to them an old person is mistreated, they don't do anything about it.

An old person doesn't have much to look forward too when they get to old to work and it just isn't right to let them stay any place where they are unhappy or where they are being mistreated.

I have planned for many years to write a book on nursing homes and try to get across to people what really goes on inside a nursing home. I have checked with other people that worked in them, and took notes and believe me my dear reader what I have told you in this book is the truth. I have not misrepresented one incident.

Oh i know many will say she has to be wrong. People aren't that cruel, but believe me my dear readers they are. This is just what goes on in a nursing home. I know it is hard to believe and I know some things I have told you seems impossible, but believe me everything I've told you is the truth.

As I have said before several nursing homes have been closed in the state of ohio because of negligence and starving the old people. But there should be more closed or else be more closely watched.

Really dear readers, something must be done about our old people and the nursing homes. As citizens of the United States it is our duty to do something and do it fast. Now don't get me wrong. I am not against nursing homes, only the way they are run. A nursing home for an old person could be something very good but as they are run today and operated my friends, they are not good.

I know if this book is published I may lose friends that are nursing home operators. But if this book will waken the people, the state, and the families, then I will feel it was written for a good cause.

As I have said before in my writing that there is a lot more to operating a nursing home than the dollar. Of course it is a business. And a profit has to be made as same as in other business but not that much profit.

Many nursing homes operators in Ohio today, and I feel it is true in other states get rich fast. Why? Because they make the money.

The wages they pay the help is the lowest. And the people they hire isn't checked out enough to know if they are eligible and yes capable of taking on the responsibility of a home full of old people. The state doesn't keep enough watch on the homes to see if they are being operated correctly. And the peoples (families) doesn't check a home good enough before placing their loved ones.

Most old people that are placed in a nursing home is capable of telling us what is going on if we would only listen. But most of us don't listen.

The old lady that I took in off the street that I told you about has a very good mind. As do many other old people her age. To me it is very sad fate when a person gets old and has nobody to care about them and no one to talk too. They are stuck in a nursing home to be abused and no one ever bothers to stop by and say a few words and just a pat on the hand. No wonder they walk and walk for what else is there for them to do. They are just like a little child. If one of us were to take a little child and put it on someone's doorstep tell me, what could it do but cry until someone came and brought it in? Then the authorities would be notified and the child would be placed in a foster home and it couldn't do a thing about it.

Well my friends, this is the same way with old people. Many have lived alone until it is impossible to do so any longer.

So many times complaints are made by the people in the community or to the family if they have one and the old person is put into a nursing home. They have to leave their homes which many have lived for many years. They have to leave behind all the pretty things that they have accumulated down through the years, gifts, furniture. Now I ask you dear readers is this not enough to make an old person go off the deep end? Then they go to a place where they don't know anyone and they have to adjust their lives. Everything is different. At the age of seventy to eighty five I can imagine that this would be very hard on them. I am sure it would be hard on us if we had to do the same thing. It's only natural the grieve for their home. Of course sometimes it can't be helped that an old person has to be put in a nursing home, if they are senile or bedfast, but let me say this to you dear readers. If an old person has a family of children and the old person was not able to stay alone but still could get around and do for themselves it would be a lot better for the children to keep their mother or father and give them a room. Let the old people be with them and the grandchildren what very short time they have left in this life. Many children grow ashamed of their parents when they get old. This too causes the old person to become despondent. This is a very sad fate. Some children say, They cause trouble. They interfere." But my dear readers we all owe our parents something.

We do owe them love respect because they are our parents. Maybe they haven't always been the best of parents but they are our parents and as a rule they loved us.

The one thing is what will our children do with us when we get old. How will we feel in our hearts and when our children tell us we have to go to a nursing home. It could happen you know.

Then when the children put this loved ones in the nursing home they seem to forget about them.

Oh, this is not true in many case but it is true in a lot of case. Some children never come at all to see them and some come just once a month to pay for them and that's it.

No wonder the old people become senile, and roam around a lot. How would one of us feel to sit all day long and wonder why our children don't come see us. Dear readers did you ever wonder what went on in an old person's mind? I have and this is what came to my mind. They Live their lives when they were well and their children all around them and in other words they live their lives over and then they wonder how it ever happen that they would end up in the nursing home. I think this too is very hard on the old people.

Then too when they are sick and become bedfast I think they understand and just give up and really don't care where they are at. I have seen this happen in many cases when they get into the nursing homes and find out how things really are inside it makes it even harder on the old person.

I know many times an old person craves something but feels it's useless to ask knowing they wouldn't get it anyway. Now tell me would it hurt the owner to buy just one little extra for a bedfast old person, or would it hurt them to devote just a little attention to the old person who has such little time left. Just the pat of a hand or a smile means a whole lot to any old person. But this is something they never get in a nursing home. Oh my dear readers it is really pitiful and sad. I am sure that if many people really knew what went on inside a nursing home. I don't think people would be so quick to put their loved ones in one of them. That is the purpose of this book is to really let the world know what really goes on in the nursing homes.

In a certain nursing home in Ohio, a very nice place and contained around thirty eight people, one of the old men became very ill. He could only be heard breathing all over the place. When the aide called the owner he was angry because he was awakened at 2AM. He came over and looked at the old man and told the aide to wait until morning and if he wasn't any better he would send him to the hospital. Around eight A.M. the old man went into a coma and they rushed him to the hospital.

Chapter 3

IN ABOUT THREE hours the old man was dead. All because the owner hated to be bothered at 2 A.M..

This often happens my dear friends. People just hate to be bothered, and old people die because of negligence on the owners part.

This same nursing home which was operated by a young couple in their twenties, bought a new car , a fire engine red convertible. Every time he got into the car to go away and she couldn't go she would go on a rampage. She would yell at the old people, also the help, She was jealous of her husband and she always felt whenever he went away alone he was going to see someone else. She would curse him to the help, yet the old people heard her. If one of them asked her anything she would yell at them and curse and this really scared the old people.

In a period of one year and a half the nursing home was closed and the old people placed in other nursing homes. These people were just too young to tie themselves down and be confined as they were. The responsibility was just too great for them.

Very often you see old people with bruises on their face and arms. If you were to ask about them the owner or aide will always say they fell, but many times this isn't true. They have been slapped. I know because I have seen this happen many, many, times.

If the owner or aide knew an old person wasn't able to walk to the bathroom alone they would say "Why isn't he walking?"

It's very hard to get around the operator of a licensed nursing home, because of two reasons. One is they have the help to lie for them, and second if the old person is rational they will be real nice to him or her until they are sure the old person has forgotten.

The help is afraid to tell the truth because they are afraid of losing their job. The old person is so glad for just a little kindness which they so very rarely get won't tell the truth either. This is the way it goes inside of a nursing home.

In the state of Ohio in 1971, a nursing home caught fire and burned up a great number of old people. In 1972, another one burned up in Cincinnati and burned up nine old people.

Now my dear readers, let's talk about these fires and the deaths of the old people. You never hear of the owner or the help getting burned up do you? Let's talk about the 1971 fire in Marietta Ohio. Where many old people were burned up. It has been said the fire could of started from someone smoking.

Well now where was the help? I have been told they had carpets on all the floors. If this is true, and some old person had dropped a cigarette on the floor or carpet, it would smoulder. If the help had been alert and checking their patients, they would seen the smoke. They are supposed to have fire extinguisher on the wall. What happen to them? How long must the fire been burning before it was noticed? Not all those old people were in one room. The fire covered many rooms and I am saying what is on my heart dear readers, that I feel if the help had been alert and doing her duties, she would of notice the fire.

She would of smelled smoke. If there were more than one person on duty, then none of them could of had their minds on there jobs. To me that was the most unnecessary thing that could happen. There absolutely was no reason why that fire should of spread into so many rooms and causing the death of so many old people. There is no excuse other than negligence. I feel that what I am saying I have a right to say. If there was faulty wiring then how come the state didn't inspect closer and often? If it was a new modern nursing home then where does the fault lay? I can't help it my friends. I know some of these old people could be saved if not all of them. There sure wasn't any speed about getting the fire department. Something is drastically wrong my friends. The same for the fire in Cincinnati Ohio.

If there is an explosion caused from the furnace and fire spreads rapidly, we can sort of understand. But when the fire is suppose to start in one room and go to many rooms and kills many people, then it is hard to understand. My opinion is it adds up to one thing. Negligence!

Now the fire in Cincinnati, as I understand it there were only ten old people. Common sense teaches you that some of those old people could of been saved. If the owners and help really cared about their old people in both fires they would of made some attempts to save the old people. You never hear of their help being written up as trying to save the old people.

It is nothing but negligence on somebody's part and if the investigation keeps probing, it will be found just where the negligence is.

But do you know my dear readers, there has not been a word mentioned about the Marietta fire until the Cincinnati fire broke out. It has been two weeks since the Cincinnati fire and that subject has died. The president of the United States was to meet the governor and the state fire marshall in the Cincinnati home. That was in the paper, but what they found out or anything else the people should know wasn't in the paper. That was the last thing that has been publicly noted about that fire. Why? There had to be a reason for those fires.

Of course has the old saying goes, It's no use to lock the barn door after the horse is out."

All the inspections and publicity won't bring those dear old people back to us. Will it?

Too many old people are dying in these nursing homes in too many odd ways. But unless they do get burned up, nothing is never done about it.

In another nursing home in Ohio which is no longer in business had a very sweet old lady. She didn't like chicken but she was given chicken any way. The owner would always give her a chicken leg. The old lady wouldn't touch it and every day, twice a day that chicken leg was warmed up and served to her. She never got any other meat until she ate that chicken leg. One day she wrapped the chicken leg up and through it into the wastebasket. The owner found it and she got a good slap in the face and wasn't allowed out of her room for a week. She never got anymore meat either. She would get two crackers for her soup. She would be so hungry she would drink the soup real fast. The crackers also would be coming back twice a day. She would get stale crackers and no bread until she ate the crackers.

 I know many of you who will read this will say no one can be that cruel to another human being, but my dear readers this is all true in a nursing home. One would never have any idea just how cruel, well , and bodied people can be to someone else who is less fortunate than they just because the other person is just a little bother and takes the well person away from his or her daily activities. It has taken me about two years to write this book and decide to publish it, but after these two nursing home fires and knowing what I know about nursing homes and what really goes on inside of one, I decided to complete this book and release it to the public. I think it is time the public really knows what goes on in these nursing homes. I do hope it will open up many eyes and something can be done about it now. Not after a big fire and lives are lost.

 I have had many old people in my home and I am known by the state, both mental and rational. I have had several people from the state hospital in Columbus, and it has not been easy because of their mentality. I have also had mental people from the government hospital in Chillicothe Ohio. But I have never hit one of them and I never used restrainers on them but one. I only tied him to a chair while waiting on the proper authorities to come and get him. Of course I have had old people from nursing homes like the old lady I took off the street. I have devoted thirty five years of my fifty six years to old people and little children. A year ago I had to give them all up because of illness. Now I have two old ladies. One I have had as I told you seven and a half years and the other lady seven years. I have never been licensed and I could only have Five, but dear readers I took those old people to drive in movies and drive in restaurants and rides in the warm summer months. Of course a business home could not do this but I am sure the owners could show a little love and compassion for their old people, don't you agree? Every Christmas Eve there was a party for my old people. The most money I ever got in all the years was one hundred and twenty five dollars an old person. Not like the nursing homes from two hundred and fifty dollars to four fifty a month. I worried over them when they were ill and if one went to the hospital. I went with them and visited them daily. It has been very confining but to me it was well worth it. I never got rich or made a lot of money. But one thing I thank God for. I have made many many old people happy for many years, If I ever do decide to have a licensed nursing home it sure will be run differently then these are today. My old people will eat and the help will have the best credentials. The pay will be enough to want the help to stay and do their job to their best of their ability.

One thing for certain dear readers if my old people don't like turkey, they'll never have to eat it. They never have and may God forbid if they ever do.

Let's pause here for a moment and really talk about disciplining an old person. You know they are like little children and can be disobedient and very rude when they want to be. But my friends does that give me the right to beat them and starve them? No it certainly doesn't. My friends do you want to know how I discipline my old people? Well I'll tell you and it has worked with most every one of mine over the period of years. If they disobey me or talk hateful to me or get angry at one another or be selfish with each other, or wet the bed, I give them a talking too in a quiet way then I won't speak to them all day. If they talk to me I wont answer them. This hurts them worse than beating or cursing at them. I tell them in a stern quite way after I shame them that until they learn to act like grown up I'm not talking to them. They'll beg me to talk to them and promise they will never be bad again if I will talk to them. After the first hour they aren't angry any longer and they are behaving. Then they start begging me to talk to them. I don't usually talk to them until about four hours after the episode. Now isn't that just like a little child? That's all old people are. My friends, just little children. Then I have no regrets that I've been mean to them. I don't say anything and no one is hurt. Do you know my dear readers in all my years of keeping old people in my home I have never had to make one old person leave. I have had some that were on their own and capable to leave without telling me until they were ready to go. When they did this, I would tell the goodbye and wish them luck. But you know something, most of them came back. I felt they would when they left. But I wanted them to be happy. I do not want anyone to stay with me if they feel they aren't happy. I know I am good to my old people and I keep most of them until God calls them home. That is the saddest part of caring for old people is dying. I miss them so terribly much after they are gone. But when they are gone I have no regrets that I ever mistreated one of them. This is my constellation and peace. If some or all of theses nursing home operators would have a little more compassion for their old people they too would have that wonder peace.

Just today I had something personal on my mind and I wasn't talking much. The two old ladies worried to death thinking that they had done something wrong. When I convinced them that they didn't, they both hugged me and told me they loved me. To me that was the highest wages that was ever been paid to me. So you see dear friends it only takes part of your hand on there's, a kind smile, and a short conversation really does wonders

Now, let's talk about how the old people are treated. The stories true. None of them are lies. THey are all true. So let's read on. There was a nursing home in Ohio who had a little old lady there, that came out to the kitchen 3 times a day. And it was always a hour after the meals.

I'm hungry when's dinner? She would say. Well one day she came out to the kitchen and she was told to go back to her room. On the way back to her room , the little old lady fell and broke her hip.

Clara Brown

The owner and a nurse ran to her . The owner too one look at her and said. Put her in bed, she is alright.

The nurse told the owner that the elderly woman's hip was broken. The owner to the nurse. There is nothing wrong with her, put her in bed and she will be alright.

Well folks, guess what happen to that poor old soul. She had to use those big stainless steel bed pans that they used to have, and that was pretty painful for that old lady.

After about a week of laying there in bed, the old lady developed a high fever. She was rushed to the hospital where she passed away.

If the owner had checked the old lady a lot better then she would have know that the old lady's hip was broken, but no the owner didn't.

One time there was this old man who had gotten into a fight with his roommate. The roommate hit the old man in the head and busted his head wide open.

The nurse told the owner that the old man needed stitches in his head.

The owner said, just put a bandage on his head and he will be alright.

The nurse asked the other nurse if she would drive her car to the hospital while she sit in the back with the old man. The nurse agreed. The owner asked, Who's going to take care of these patients if you take him to the hospital? Then you call the squad for him. The nurse said. Oh no! I can't do that, that will give this home a bad name.

The old man had to have 5 stitches put in his head. But the owner was more interested in getting a bad name then she was the old man.

Then there was a man who was only 48 yrs . Old who was in a nursing home for rehab. He was a very big man. He weighed about 300 pounds. His wife came out to see and he was crying . His wife asked him why was he crying for?

This man couldn't talk so he pointed down at his stomach. His wife lifted up his heavy stomach and it was all blood raw. Parts of it was bleeding. His wife asked him what happen.

When the nurse came in to give him a bath, she had scrubbed

under his stomach so hard that it started to bleed. The nurse didn't care that she had gotten it to bleed, she just left the room without putting any medicine on it.

The wife got mad. She went down to the nursing station and put in a complaint. The head nurse went and found out which nurse that gave the man his bath. And brought her back to his room and asked the patient if she was the one that gave him his bath, and he said yes. His wife jumped all over the nurse and told her that she was never to take care of her husband again. So the head nurse took her out to through the door and had a talk with her. Instead of the head nurse firing the nurse, she put the nurse at the other end of the floor and the nurse did the same thing to another patient and it was there between both wives they got the nurse fired and now she isn't allowed to work around any Patients at all.

Now friends, why didn't the head nurse fire the nurse? Why did she give the nurse a chance to do it again? Maybe she was friends away from the nursing home. Why was another patient have to be hurt in the prosse? I don't know.

There was this old man in his eighties. The nurse had put him on the pot and then forgot about him. He sat there for a long time, soon his bottom started to hurt him so he got up and tried to get to his bed but he fell on the floor and hit his head. The lady who delivered the food trays went to take his tray in and found him on the floor.

She called for the nurse's but the nurse didn't come. She called them for 45 minutes and the nurse's still didn't come. She had to go to the nurse's station to get a nurse. The nurses were sitting there laughing and was having a really good time. The tray person told the nurse's that there was a patient on the floor and he needed help stat. She also told them that if they didn't get down there stat that she was going to have all of their jobs. The nurses took off and went to the room. But when the head nurse and tray person got there the head nurse started to yell at the old person for trying to walk without help the tray person looked at the head nurse and told her that if someone was paying attention to the call light and gotten him up and back in bed he would not have even tried to do it by himself in the first place and to stop yelling at him like he is a low life because he is the one that pays their wages. When the tray person got back to the kitchen and she was so mad that she told her boss about it and her boss gave her a complaint paper two days later the same tray person and the same floor again went past the station and notice that there was all new different people there she asked, where are the regular nurses? Guess what happen? They told her that the other nurses had been fired because of a tray passenger. That really made the tray person really happy no one abuse a patient around her.

Now friends, why wasn't the nurses doing their jobs that they were getting paid for. Do you feel the tray person done the right thing? I sure do.

The old man was lucky because the tray passer had them all fired.

There was an old man who didn't do as the nurse told him to do so the nurse had the orderly to beat him. The orderly really beat him so hard that the old man almost died.

Did the orderly or the nurse get fired? No they didn't. They got away with it. They said the old man had fallen.

Why did the orderly listen to the nurse and why wasn't they both fired? What was the owner thinking about when he didn't fire them both.

In one nursing home in Ohio, there was a little old lady. Every night these two orderly's (who were on drugs) would go into the old lady's room and pull the hair out on the lady's private parts then laugh about it when she would cry out in pain. Every night they would do that to the poor old lady. Another orderly then came into the room and caught them and turned the in. Why didn't the owner have them checked out before they were hired, but no they didn't.

In one nursing home, where a woman was in there for rehab. The nursing home had cats there too. The cats were allowed to roam the nursing home. The cats were covered with fleas so bad that the fleas were getting on the beds and the patients. The lady told her family that she couldn't sleep at night for the fleas biting on her.

The Inside Truth About Nursing Homes

How was she able to get well if she couldn't get her rest? Cats are great but not in a nursing home if they are full of fleas?

In one nursing home, they would take the wet draw sheet off of the patient bed and instead of washing the draw sheet, they would hang them up in the bathroom to dry. Then they would put them back on the patient bed.

Now friends, would you lay on a dirty draw sheet? No you wouldn't but those old people had too.

The nursing home had a real bad smell to it. Those poor old people had to smell that everyday.

There was one nurse who wouldn't put the dirty draw sheets back under the patients. She would always put clean draw sheet on the patient bed. She got fired for it.

There was this one nursing home were this one nurse had been doing nursing for many, many years. She knew a lot about nursing but her supervisor had just got out of nursing school and she didn't know to much about nursing. Only what she learned in nursing school.

One day a patient got sick, very sick. So the nurse who knew about nursing told the new supervisor what she would do for the old lady, the supervisor got mad and she fired the nurse. Now friends, why didn't the supervisor talk to the nurse instead if firing the nurse. You know friends, there are a few nurses who take the patients welfare at heart but there are not many of them who don't.

One night a nurse was taking a elderly woman up stairs to bed and just because the old lady was slow getting up stairs, the owner came up and hit the old lady.

Now don't do that Honey, that hurt. The old lady said.

The nurse told the owner that she will take her up stairs by herself. The owner walked away.

In one nursing home, there was a woman who was very sick. She couldn't feed herself or do one thing for herself. Her two daughters came out to see her that evening. When they got to their mothers room what they saw made them so mad that they could bite a nail into. Well folks are you ready for this? The woman was put there the day before. When they gave her a shot, they had gotten some blood on her sheets.

When her two daughters got there around 4:30 P.M. Their mother still had the same sheets on her bed with the blood on them. She had not had her bath and clean sheets put on her bed and her breakfast tray was still in front of her and her food was very cold. She had coffee all over her. Boy, the two daughters got so mad to see their mother in that bad shape that they stormed down to the nurses station. All the nurses were standing around and laughing and having a wonderful time.

Chapter 4

THE TWO DAUGHTERS had to hollow at them to get their attention.

We will call this lady Mrs. Smith.

We are Mrs. Smith daughters. She is in room 112 and we want our mother to have a hot meal brought to her and we want her to have a bath and clean gown put on her now!

We will get to her when we can. One nurse said. You will get to her now or we will have all of you fired.

Boy, you should have seen the nurses run around to get to Mrs. Smith taken care of. The nurses had a hot meal brought to her, she had a bath and a clean gown put on her.

I want my mother hand fed until she is able to feed herself. Do you hear me? One daughter said.

Yes, I heard you.

And another thing, nurse, if I ever come out here and see my mother in this shape again, then I'll have you all fired from your jobs.

Yes Ma'am, the nurse said.

Now my friends, those nurse's couldn't do enough for Mrs. Smith.

When Mrs. Smith got better, then her daughters took their mother home.

The one daughter took her mother home with her and took good care of her until Mrs. Smith passed away and that was years later.

Now friends, It was all uncalled for the nurses to be threaten to lose their jobs if they had been doing their jobs in the first place, but they thought it was more important to have fun then to take care of their patients.

Friends, would you like to be treated like Mrs. Smith was treated or like these other old people in this book was treated? No you wouldn't . Would you like to have your parents treated like that? No you wouldn't. If you love your parents, then you wouldn't want them being treated like these old people were treated.

You would think that these nursing homes would be better than the old homes that I had worked in, but the old people are treated a little better but not much.

The old people are still treated badly.

Folks, we need to do something to stop the old people from being treated the way that they are treated.

I've talked to some people that has worked in these newer homes and they told me alot about how the old people are treated.

It is so sad.

These old people has feelings and all they want is for someone to love them and be good to then that is all.

If I had my parents with me then I would take care of them and love them.

Dad died January 18, 1952 but mom spent the last week at my house when she died. I never raised my voice at her. I took real good care of her. I had promised my mother that she wouldn't go to a nursing home and folks, she didn't go to one.

When our parents was raising their kids, they had to do without for us, and they had to stay home and lose out on a lot of fun because of their kids, so why can't we do that for our parents instead of putting them in a nursing home just because they tie us down.

We don't want to take the time to take care of them like they did us.

My friends, just stop and think about it.

They took care of us so let's take care of them your parents being treated that way.

The Inside Truth About Nursing Homes

I talked to my granddaughter. She had worked in one of the new nursing home and this is what she told me that she saw how the patients were treated. The old people was slapped up a side the head, and if the old person was to raise their hand to protect their self then the nurse would twist the old persons finger.

If the old person asked for a glass of water or a snack, then they would not get it.

If the patient wet the bed or mess the bed, then they had to lay in it. If they asked to have a bath, then they wouldn't get it.

My friends, would you want your parents to be treated that way? I don't think so, neither would I want my parents to be treated that way.

Folks, there was this one nursing home in Ohio, that had this old lady who couldn't stretch out her legs. The nurse was putting the old ladys pants on her. The nurse was having a hard time putting the pants on the old lady.

So the nurse finally that if she pressed down on the old ladys legs and straighten the legs out then the pants would go on easy. She started pressing down on the legs. It took just a few minutes of pushing down on the legs to cause the legs to break.

Was the nurse fired? No she wasn't.

She gotta stay there and worked, but the poor old lady had two broken legs.

Now friends, Tell me what is wrong with this picture? The nurse should of been fired so she couldn't do that to another old person.

I was told yesterday that this woman in Ohio that had her father in a nursing home.

The man was up in years and he couldn't walk good by himself.

Well, he had to go to the bathroom, so he called the nurse to come and take him to the bathroom.

The nurse said she would be right in , but she never came. The man waited and waited but the nurse never came. So the man got up out of his chair and started walking to the bathroom.

When he got to the bathroom door, he fell and hit his head on the dresser. He was out cold and his head was bleeding.

They rushed him to the hospital and the next day he passed away.

When his daughter tried to found out what happen, no one would tell her anything of what happened to him. She even asked the doctor and he wouldn't tell her anything. Even today she doesn't know what happen to her dad.

You know my friends, they could have told her what happen to her dad, but instead she had to found out for herself.

She didn't tell me how she found out the truth about her dad.

Well friends, you tell me, what is wrong with this picture? Why didn't the nursing home or the doctor tell the woman what happen to her dad.

Today, I was told this old woman that her mother was in a nursing home. Her dad had died in October so in November at Thanksgiving, She brought her mother home to spend some time with her. Her mother got very sick while she was there. She stated to get sick to her stomach and throwing up. The daughter said that her mother's vomit smilt like bowels. She took her mother back to the nursing home. She told the home to get the Doctor out there to see her mother. They told her that the Doctor was out there and her vitals were just fine. When the daughter went back out to see her mother, she heard her mother hollow, Please help me, somebody please help me, I'm in so much pain, Please help me.

The nurses just walked by her mothers room and didn't even go into to see what was wrong. The daughter went and took her mother to the hospital. At the hospital, they found out that her mother had cancer and cancer had eaten up most of her mother's insides. Her mother died that night.

Folks, why didn't the nurses notice that something was wrong with her mother? Why didn't the doctor notice that her mother's vitals signs were way down.

There are many Ways but no answers.

Another woman told me her mother was in a nursing home in Ohio. She was there for rehab. She went to see her mother. When she got there they had her mother up in a chair. She had been in the chair all day. The nurses had not been in the to see about her. Er mother was in alot of pain and she was tired from sitting there all day that she was crying. Her daughter asked her mother why she was crying? I've been sitting here all day and I;m in alot of pain.

Has the nurse been in to see about you Mom? No, I haven't seen no one all day only when they brought my dinner and supper. The nurses hasn't been in all day.

Well the daughter got real mad about it and called her brother and told him about their mother. He got real mad too and he went to the nursing home. He told the nurses off and took his mother out of that nursing home. His mother never had to go to another nursing home again.

Well folks, I've told you what really goes on in these nursing homes.

We really don't want to be treated like all of these old people that you read about in this book.

It is very sad to know how these old people are treated.

My mother never had to go to a nursing home and my daughter said that I would never have to go to one. I'm very glad about that.

Now a days they have Home Care nursing. People who will come to your house to care of your loved ones.

Just stop and think before you put your loved ones away in a nursing home.

I have seen it all and the whole truth. None of the are lies.

I've seen it and a lot of people who had loved ones in the nursing homes have told me what happen to their parents when they were in these places told me what happen to the old people.

My mother and I both worked in nursing homes and we saw a lot of bad things in these places.

I'm glad I'm too old and not able to do nursing again.

Now the nursing homes today are better than they were back then. They have cleaning people to do the cleaning, have men to do the heavy lifting, they have the barber to cut the men's hair and the beauty polar to do the women's hair and the nurses just take care of the patients. But still the nurses doesn't do their jobs right.

Clara Brown

One man in a nursing home has something wrong with his eye, two ladies came to visit. When they saw his eye, the ladies told the main nurse about it. She said she would take care of it. A month later the same two ladies came and visit the man. They asked him if he had seen an eye doctor yet and he said no. The man was in his fifties and he had his right mind. He had had 2 strokes and couldn't use his left side, and that is what he was in there.

Now why didn't the nursing home have his eyes checked out? The nurses says that he refused to be checked out. But we know that isn't the truth. The two ladies told him that he could go blind if he don't have it checked out so he promised that he would. We will see by next month.

There was another man in one of our todays nursing home.

His daughter came out to see him. He was swollen so bad he couldn't even get his breath.

She told the nurses off and took her dad to the hospital. The hospital kept him for a week. They had taken 6 liters of fluid off of him. The daughter moved him out of that nursing home and into another nursing home. She isn't able to take care of him herself.

The nursing home wants to charge this man five thousand and two hundred dollars for him to stay there.

Now tell me my friends, who can afford to pay that much money? I can't, can you?

The man is in his right mind. He wants to come home to his own home but there is noone there to care of him.

This nursing home even asked him if he had any house that they could sell. He told them all he had was his home and he wasn't going to sell it.

These nursing homes wants to strip their patients down to where the patients has nothing left.

That is very wrong.

I know that the nursing homes has to pay all of the workers and all, but to take everything that a patient has is very wrong.

Folks, one day we'll be old and wouldn't you want to be treated the way that these old people are treated.

No we wouldn't. I am 75 years old now and my daughter says I will never go to a nursing home. I am glad about that.

My mother spent her last days on this earth living at my home and she never did.

There will come a time my friends, when every one of us will be old just like these old people in this book. Have any of you ever stopped to think what will happen to you when you get old and can not take care of yourself.

There was this elderly lady who was in a nursing home in Springfield, Ohio. I knew this lady a long time so when i heard about this elderly woman being mistreated, I had to write about it.

Just because this lady had wet herself, the nurse would give her water from the bathroom instead of giving her ice water like they did the other patients. Why didn't they give ice water to her. They would also slap her around a lot, and they would not go in to check on her like they were suppose too. Also when the night nurse forgot to give this lady her medicine for the night so in the morning they double her medicine that next morning and this poor old lady died.

In another nursing home in Springfield, Ohio, the nurses was cleaning the old man's teeth. She dropped the teeth and broke them. The nursing home was going to make this old man pay to get the teeth fixed. He had to threaten to call his lawyer, then the nursing home agree to pay to have the teeth fixed.

Now, was this right? Why didn't they just go ahead and have them fixed? *Instead of getting the old man upset and threaten them. The old people don't have a fighting chance against the nursing homes and how they are treated.*

In another nursing home in Ohio there was this old lady. Another patient ran over this old lady's foot with his wheelchair. The patients in the wheelchair was a big person. When the second person ran over the lady's foot, it caused the foot to break open pretty bad. The nurse did bandage the foot up but the nurse would only change the bandage every four or five days. The old lady almost lost her foot. The nursing

Clara Brown

home didn't even take the old lady to the hospital. That poor old soul could have lost her foot, but the nursing home didn't care. All they thought about wa the money that the poor old soul was paying.

In a lot of the nursing homes they have patients sitting in wheelchairs in the lobbies. These old people are sitting half in their wheelchair and half out of their wheelchairs.

You know just by looking at them that they are not comfortable sitting like that. Why want the nurses sit them back up to where they are comfortable.

I have been in alot of nursing homes and I see a lot of it.

The nurse's just walk past them and keep right on going. They don't stop and straighten the old people in the chair so that the poor old soul could be more comfortable sitting there.

In a nursing home, there was an old lady who was bed fast. She had had a stroke the one side of her body was paralyzed. These two orderly's was working and when no one was around or near by, these two orderly's guys would rape this poor old soul. They told her that if she told anyone then they would kill her family. That poor old soul was afraid to say anything to anyone. She didn't want her family to get hurt, so she kept her mouth shut, But one nurse did over hear the two orderly's talk about the old lady, and they were talking about going to her room and raping her again. The nurse said nothing but she did watch the two boys and when they went to the old lady's room. They went in to rape her, but the poor old soul was dead. The boys didn't know she was dead so they went ahead and raped her. The nurse caught caught them in the act, The boys threatened to hurt her family if she told anyone. She didn't tell a soul. The boys quit their jobs. Nothing was said about the boys. But ten years later the boys was killed in a car accident so nothing was done about it and it was told to the family then to me. The police couldn't do nothing about it becaused the old lady was dead and so wasn;t the boy's.

In one nursing home in Ohio, a woman went to see an elderly woman. The woman was pretty old. She was laying across her bed with the sides rails up. She was very uncomfortable laying that way.

The Inside Truth About Nursing Homes

The woman who came to see the elderly woman and asked her if she was comfortable and the elderly woman said no. The woman straighten her up in bed and asked her if she was comfortable now? The elderly woman said yes and she Thanked the woman.

The nurses would walk by her room but would never stopped in to see about her. A outsider had to do the job of the nurses.

One woman went to go see her husband in a nursing home, and her husband had a tray of cold food sitting there. She asked her husband why didn't he eat his dinner? Because when i touch the fork it shocks me. He said.

How does a fork shock you honey?

THe bed is up against the outlet and the outlet is bad. I can't even touch my side railings it will shock me. Told the nurses but they won't do anything about it. The wife went and told the nurses. There's nothing we can do about it, the nurse said.

The wife asked about the maintenance man?

Well he is a busy, the nurse said.

The wife told the nurse off then went back to her husband. She pulled the bed away from the wall so her husband wouldn't get shocked. Then she told the nurse she wanted a tray of hot food for her husband or she was going to have the nursing home closed down. Her husband got the hot food.

Now folks, now wouldn't it have been a whole lot better if the nurse would have gotten the maintenance man to come and fix the light socket, But no, the nurse wouldn't do it.

That light socket could have caused a fire and a lot of old people would have burned up in that fire. What do we have to do to get the nurses to put the old peoples welfare at heart.

These old people should come first with the nurses. After all, it's the old people who pays the wages to the nurses. Without the old peoples money then the nurses wouldn't get paid.

There was a old man in a nursing home in Ohio, The man was very stubborn. He didn't like being told what to do. One day the nurse went into the mans room.

Clara Brown

Okay Mr. Smith (Name made up) time to get up.

I don't feel like getting up this morning, He said. I just want to lay here in bed. Mr. Smith said.

The nurse spoke up. You're getting up today even tho you don't want to.

But I don't feel to good today, please Let me stay in bed. Mr. Smith begged.

The nurse made him get up out of bed. He was put into the chair and the nurse tied him down to the chair.

Why are you tying me down for? Mr. Smith asked.

So you wouldn't go back to bed when my back is turned. the nurse said.

You don't tell me what to do. I don't take orders from you. The old man said. I'm going back to bed, I'm sick, I need to lay down.

No you are not going back to bed, your going to sit there all day, The nurse said as she slapped the old man in the face. Then the nurse walked out of the room.

The old man hollowed all day, I'm sick, I want to lay down. That went on all day. The nurse didn't pay any attention to that poor old soul.

That night when the night nurse came on duty, the old man was in pretty bad shape. He died the next morning.

When the day trick nurse came on duty. She went to his room to get him up. The bed was empty. Where is Mr. Smith? The nurse asked the another nurse.

Oh, Mr. Smith died early this morning. The nurse said.

Well at least we don't have to sit and listen to him screaming like he did yesterday.

Well folks, That nurse was just working for is Quitting time and pay day. She didn't have the welfare of the patients at heart.

Chapter 5

IN ONE NURSING home a nurse stole 3 pocket books that belongs to 3 elderly ladies. When the ladies found their purses gone, they asked everyone if they had seen their purses.

These poor old souls was hurt. They lost the pictures of their loved ones, their money, just everything.

Well folks, There is no since in someone stealing those poor old souls purses. Why not steal from someone who don't have much, why not steal from people who has something. But on the other hand, why steal at all.

Well folks, these old people don't have a fighting chance in these nursing homes. They are either getting slapped or have their thing stolen from them. I really feel sorry for them. Don't you?

In another nursing home , there was this little old lady that had Alzheimer's. THe nursing home was very mean to this old lady. When the family found out how she was treated, they took her out of that nursing home and put her into another nursing home. At the new nursing home,they just let her do whatever she wanted to do. This can be dangerous. The old lady could go roaming threw the nursing home and end up somewhere that she shouldn't be at, like in the kitchen around the stove or maybe in the basement around the furnace.

They should have kept a close eye on her, but they didn't.

How many old people have to go threw with torement and abuse that they have to go threw in what few years that they have left to live? Why do they have to be abuse? Why not give them some love instead of being mistreated?

Now let's talk about the married couples that goes to these nursing homes.

These people have been together for 40 or 50 years or more. But as soon as they are put in a nursing home, then they are seperated.

The husband is put in one room and the wife is put in another room far from her husband.

Now folks, is this right? Why can't they have a room together? Let them spend the rest of their lives together. It would make them very happy. And the nurses gets upset when they have to go to another room to give the patient their medication and sometimes they get even with that patient when they are alone by yelling at them or even hitting on them.

Now let's talk about when a patient is dying. Does a nursing home call the family when their love ones is dying? No they don't.

They wait until the patient has died, then they call the family. The family don't even get to say their goodbyes to their love ones.

As soon as they see a patient is dying, that is when they should call the family. That way the family can say their goodbyes to them.

In one nursing home, a patient came into a nursing home and had head lice. They thought that the wife had gave them to him. But it wasn't the wife who gave them to him, it was his sister that gave them to him.

His wife had to stand at the door and talk to her husband. She couldn't even hold his hand. His sister was allowed to go into his room and hug him whenever she wanted too, but not his wife. His wife was very hurt over this. She knew she didn't have head lice and she didn't know that he had them until the nurse told her. Finally, one day she was talking to her sister-in law about the head lice. His sister reply was, Oh I'm going to have to give myself a treatment before I go out there to see him again. I didn't know I gave them to him.

The man's wife got very upset when her sister-in law told her that she had them. The wife told the nurses and the nurses wouldn't let his sister back into see him. The wife and the sister-in law had to take a treatments at the health department before they could go see him again. They should have checked the his wife's head before saying anything so mean to her. It caused her husband to get very upset. And he was wanting to go home because of the way his wife was being treated. They could have done it in a different way so that they could keep the old man calmed.

Why didn't the nurses get onto it as soon as they found out about the head lice? Why because they didn't want to take the time to do anything.

Now I will say this about nursing homes. There are a few of them that is really nice and the patients are given very good care of, but even today there is is some nursing homes that is still very mean to the patients.

In one nursing home a very close friend of mine was in a nursing home. I went out to see her. I asked her how she was doing?

Oh, I'm so mad right now that I could bite a nail into, she said.

Now folks, this lady still had her right mind and I knew her since I was a baby. She even put diapers on me. That's how long I have knew her. We were very close.

Well honey, what got you so upset? I asked her.

I haven't had my bath or my hair washed for a week. I asked them when I was going to get a bath? The nurse said whenever we can get to you.

I went to find the nurse.

Look nurse, my friend hasn't had a bath in a week. Now I want her to have a bath and her head washed today or I'm going to have you all fired and I'll have this nursing home shut down. Now do you hear me nurse?

Yes I hear you but I don't have the time right now.

Alright, I'll just have you fired, and I'll have this place closed down by tomorrow. I said.

Clara Brown

I'll do it right now, the nurse said.

My friends husband and I stayed there until my friend had her bath and her hair washed.

When the nurse came back into the room with her, I told the nurse, Now she better have her bath everyday, do you hear me nurse?

Yes I hear you. The nurse said.

When I go out to see my friend, she would have her bath and her hair washed. She was very happy that she got her bath everyday.

It was told to me today this this woman's father was in a nursing home. The nurse took his clothes and gave the clothes to another man in the nursing home. She asked the nurse what happen to her father's clothes. The nurse just walked right out of the room and not saying even one word. Now, you all know that it was the nurse that should have answered the woman's question and told her the truth. It wasn't right the way the patient or the family was treated too.

What would have you all done if this was your parent and you found someone else wearing your parents clothes?

Now let me tell you something, folks. If that had been my father and I seen another man wear my dad's shirt, I would raise all kind of cain with the nursing home.

As the lady got ready to go home, she was walking down the hall when she saw another man wearing her father's shirt. She knew the shirt because it was the one that she had gotten it for him at christmas time.

When she asked the nurse about it, the nurse just turned around and walked away.

In another nursing home, there was this old lady and her husband. They both were put in the same room together. They both had alzheimer's disease.

One day the man pulled his wife's hair so the nursing home put them both in separate rooms. The husband was asking about how his wife was doing and they kept telling him that she had died but yet she was still alive. One day the lady fell and broke her hip. They put her in bed and told the husband that wife had died. The husband didn't *go to see his wife again because he thought she was dead. She died a week later, Because she wasn't given the proper care when she fell and broke her hip.*

I was also told this morning that a woman was talking to the nurse and said that she had to go to the bathroom. The nurse told her to get up off of her lazy butt and go to the bathroom by herself.

Well folks, Now let me tell you something about this poor old soul. She could walk but she had to have help. This nurse knew that but she didn't care for this poor old lady.

The poor old woman tried to get up to go to the bathroom. She fell and broke her hip. She laid on the floor for awhile . She hollered for help but noone came to help her.

When they finally did get to her, she was in very bad shape. Her hip was broken.

The nurse just put her in her bed and just left her there. They didn't call the squad to get her to the hospital. They just put her in bed and just forgotten about her. The next morning they went into her room and found her dead.

Now tell me something folk, Why didn't that nurse help the lady to the bathroom and why did the nurse get so hateful with her? When the lady called for help, then why didn't they come to help her? Also, why did the nurse just put the lady in bed then leave her there? Why didn't the nurse call the ambulance and have her taken to the hospital?

This was told to me tonight.

This lady went over to see her mother when she got off of work. She didn't know how sick her mother really was until she got there. She called her family and asked they would just come over for a few hours a day to help her to take care of mother. Noone wanted to help her out so she had to put her mother in a nursing home.

The first few months, the family came to see her.

Then they started to slack off. They wrote letters but they started to slack off too.

One day, the lady asked where her mother clothes were at? The nurse said she had no idea where the clothes were at but they would

Clara Brown

look into it, but nothing happen.

They told her, her mother was doing good but that was wrong too.

When you visit someone in a nursing home, you only see the outside of them and not the outside of them.

This is what the nursing home hid from the daughter.

She went out to see her mother one day and the nursing had her mother in a wheelchair. When she asked about that, they reply, It's for her own safety. As time went by her mother would never walk. She asked the nursing home why they wasn't getting her mother up to walking. They always said that her mother didn't want to walk.

She watched her mother go from laughing, smiling, talking to doing nothing. The changes was really beginning to show up on her mother.

The family had stopped coming to see her.

One day, the daughter went to see her mother and notice her mother wasn't talking very good. If you asked her something, she would say um um. When she would eat, she would do a lot of coughing.

The home said her mother would not drink her water. Folks, this poor old soul could not do anything for herself. The nursing home had to do everything for her. Like bathing, taking her to the bathroom.

Folks, if you do not go and see your loved ones in the nursing homes, you don't know the hell that they go threw.

If the daughter missed a few days of getting out to see her mother, then when she did get out to see her, she could tell her mother had not been taking care of. Her mother's clothes smelled like a goat, Her feet and legs were raw from the pee and bowels running down her legs.

Her mother went threw 3 roommates that died in less than 6 months.

It took a toll on her mother. When she asked the Doctor about it. The doctor said that was Normal.

In no time, her mother was bed fast. She was in and out of the hospital.

The staff would bring her a tray of food knowing that she couldn't feed herself. They would not feed her. They told the daughter that her *mother did not want to eat.*

The mother could not turn herself in bed. When they finally would turn her, she would scream out in pain. Her feet stink because of the gang green on her feet. Her feet looked like they were rotten. She had thrash in her mouth and on the outside of her mouth.

The nursing home had kept her mother in one spot for 3 ½ days at a time. When they did turn her or try to turn her, her body was frozen in a fetal position. Finally the mother passed away.

Folks, when a person is treated that way, it is all uncall for. There is no sense in it. Be careful where you put your love ones and Please, Please, Please go and see them . Don't forget about them.

Will you end up in a nursing home and being mistreated like these old people are being treated. Will you have everything that you worked so hard to get, being taken away from you?

Think about it folks, Think long and hard about it.

Will your kids take care of you when you get old or will they just throw you away into a nursing home and forget about you.

Well folks, I wish you all the luck in the world when you get old.

God Bless you all.

                                        Signed By,
                            Mary F. Brake and Clara L. Brown

www.ingramcontent.com/pod-product-compliance
Lightning Source LLC
Chambersburg PA
CBHW050026230526
45470CB00003B/1153